The Perfect Dash Diet

The Cooking Guide For Every Beginner

Candace Hickman

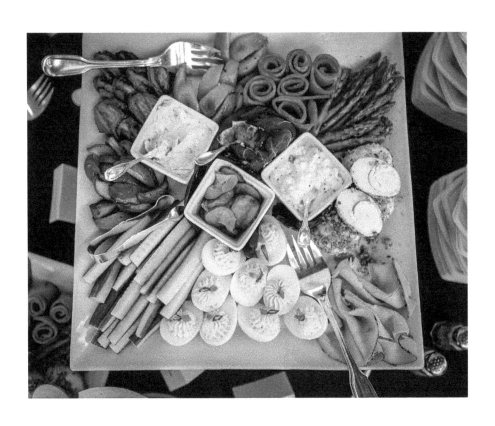

TABLE OF CONTENT

6

Chickpeas Stew

Preparation time: 10 minutes

Cooking time: 20 minutes

Servings: 4

Ingredients:

- 1 tablespoon olive oil
- 1 yellow onion, chopped
- 2 teaspoons chili powder
- 14 ounces canned chickpeas, no-salt-added, drained and rinsed
- 14 ounces canned tomatoes, no-salt-added, cubed
- 1 cup low-sodium chicken stock
- 1 tablespoon cilantro, chopped
- A pinch of black pepper

Directions:

1. Heat up a pot with the oil over medium-high heat, add the onion and chili powder, stir and cook for 5 minutes.
2. Add the chickpeas and the other ingredients, toss, cook for 15 minutes over medium heat, divide into bowls and serve for lunch.

Nutrition info per serving: 425 calories, 20.7g protein, 67.3g carbohydrates, 9.9g fat, 19.5g fiber, 0mg cholesterol, 77mg sodium, 1170mg potassium

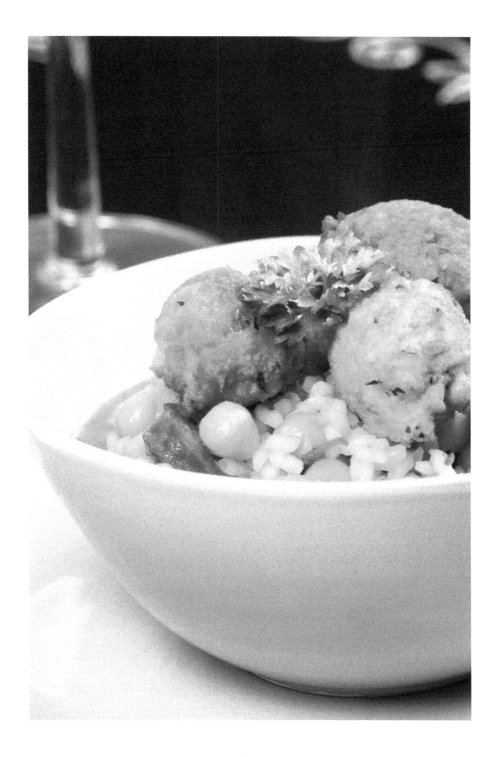

Lemon Chicken Salad

Preparation time: 10 minutes

Cooking time: 0 minutes

Servings: 4

Ingredients:

- 1 tablespoon olive oil
- A pinch of black pepper
- 2 rotisserie chicken, skinless, boneless, shredded
- 1 pound cherry tomatoes, halved
- 1 red onion, chopped
- 4 cups baby spinach
- ¼ cup walnuts, chopped
- ½ teaspoon lemon zest, grated
- 2 tablespoons lemon juice

Directions:

1. In a salad bowl, combine the chicken with the tomato and the other ingredients, toss and serve for lunch.

Nutrition info per serving: 199 calories, 21.6g protein, 10.6g carbohydrates, 9.1g fat, 3.2g fiber, 53mg cholesterol, 292mg sodium, 527mg potassium

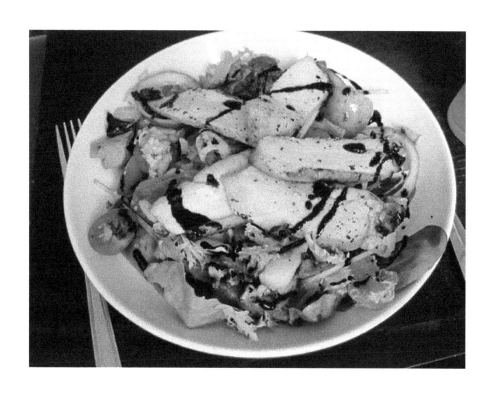

Asparagus Salad

Preparation time: 10 minutes

Cooking time: 20 minutes

Servings: 4

Ingredients:

- 3 garlic cloves, minced
- 2 tablespoons olive oil
- 1 red onion, chopped
- 3 carrots, sliced
- ½ cup low-sodium chicken stock
- 2 cups baby spinach
- 1 pound asparagus, trimmed and halved
- 1 red bell pepper, cut into strips
- 1 yellow bell pepper, cut into strips
- 1 green bell pepper, cut into strips
- A pinch of black pepper

Directions:

1. Heat up a pan with the oil over medium-high heat, add the onion and the garlic, stir and sauté for 2 minutes.
2. Add the asparagus and the other ingredients except the spinach, toss, and cook for 15 minutes.

3. Add the spinach, cook everything for 3 minutes more, divide into bowls and serve for lunch.

Nutrition info per serving: 141 calories, 4.7g protein, 17.8g carbohydrates, 7.4g fat, 5.9g fiber, 0mg cholesterol, 66mg sodium, 669mg potassium

Tomato Beef Stew

Preparation time: 10 minutes

Cooking time: 1 hour and 20 minutes

Servings: 4

Ingredients:

- 1 pound beef stew meat, cubed
- 1 cup no-salt-added tomato sauce
- 1 cup low-sodium beef stock
- 1 tablespoon olive oil
- 1 yellow onion, chopped
- ¼ teaspoon hot sauce
- 1 teaspoon onion powder
- 1 teaspoon garlic powder
- 1 tablespoon cilantro, chopped

Directions:

1. Heat up a pot with the oil over medium-high heat, add the meat and the onion, stir and brown for 5 minutes.
2. Add the tomato sauce and the rest of the ingredients, bring to a simmer and cook over medium heat for 1 hour and 15 minutes.
3. Divide into bowls and serve for lunch.

Nutrition info per serving: 273 calories, 36.2g protein, 6.9g carbohydrates, 10.7g fat, 1.6g fiber, 101mg cholesterol, 440mg sodium, 715mg potassium

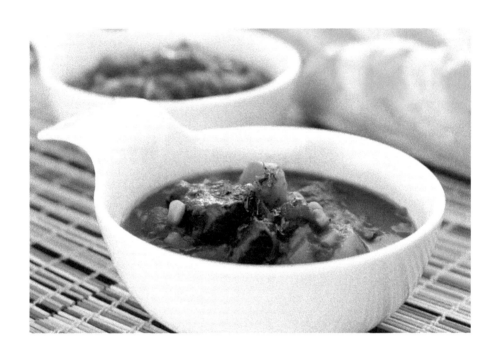

Rosemary Pork Chops

Preparation time: 5 minutes

Cooking time: 8 hours and 10 minutes

Servings: 4

Ingredients:

- 4 pork chops
- 1 tablespoon olive oil
- 2 shallots, chopped
- 1 pound white mushrooms, sliced
- ½ cup low-sodium beef stock
- 1 tablespoon rosemary, chopped
- ¼ teaspoon garlic powder
- 1 teaspoon sweet paprika

Directions:

1. Heat up a pan with the oil over medium-high heat, add the pork chops and the shallots, toss, brown for 10 minutes and transfer to a slow cooker.
2. Add the rest of the ingredients, put the lid on and cook on Low for 8 hours.
3. Divide the pork chops and mushrooms between plates and serve for lunch.

Nutrition info per serving: 324 calories, 22.2g protein, 6.4g carbohydrates, 23.9g fat, 1.7g fiber, 69mg cholesterol, 82mg sodium, 692mg potassium

Balsamic Shrimp Salad

Preparation time: 10 minutes

Cooking time: 8 minutes

Servings: 4

Ingredients:

- 1 tablespoon olive oil
- 1 red onion, sliced
- 1 pound shrimp, peeled and deveined
- 2 cups baby arugula
- 1 tablespoon balsamic vinegar
- 1 tablespoon lemon juice
- 1 tablespoon coriander, chopped
- A pinch of black pepper

Directions:

1. Heat up a pan with the oil over medium heat, add the onion, stir and sauté for 2 minutes.
2. Add the shrimp and the other ingredients, toss, cook for 6 minutes, divide into bowls and serve for lunch.

Nutrition info per serving: 180 calories, 26.4g protein, 4.8g carbohydrates, 5.6g fat, 0.8g fiber, 239mg cholesterol, 282mg sodium, 278mg potassium

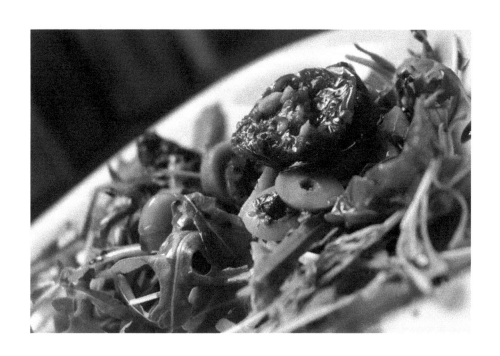

Eggplant and Tomato Stew

Preparation time: 5 minutes

Cooking time: 20 minutes

Servings: 4

Ingredients:

- 1 pound eggplants, roughly cubed
- 2 garlic cloves, minced
- 2 tablespoons olive oil
- 1 yellow onion, chopped
- 1 teaspoon sweet paprika
- ½ cup cilantro, chopped
- 14 ounces low-sodium canned tomatoes, chopped
- 1 tablespoon cilantro, chopped

Directions:

1. Heat up a pan with the oil over medium-high heat, add the onion and the garlic and sauté for 2 minutes.
2. Add the eggplant and the other ingredients except the cilantro, bring to a simmer and cook for 18 minutes.
3. Divide into bowls and serve with the cilantro sprinkled on top.

Nutrition info per serving: 153 calories, 2.9g protein, 18.4g carbohydrates, 8.6g fat, 6.2g fiber, 3mg cholesterol, 35mg sodium, 329mg potassium

Beef and Scallions Mix

Preparation time: 10 minutes

Cooking time: 30 minutes

Servings: 4

Ingredients:

- 1 and ¼ cups low-sodium beef stock
- 1 yellow onion, chopped
- 1 tablespoon olive oil
- 2 cups peas
- 1 pound beef stew meat, cubed
- 1 cup canned tomatoes, no-salt-added and chopped
- 1 cup scallions, chopped
- ¼ cup parsley, chopped
- Black pepper to the taste

Directions:

1. Heat up a pot with the oil over medium-high heat, add the onion and the meat and brown for 5 minutes.
2. Add the peas and the other ingredients, stir, bring to a simmer and cook over medium heat for 25 minutes more.
3. Divide the mix into bowls and serve for lunch.

Nutrition info per serving: 331 calories, 41.2g protein, 16.9g carbohydrates, 11.1g fat, 5.6g fiber, 101mg cholesterol, 131mg sodium, 870mg potassium

Lime Turkey Stew

Preparation time: 5 minutes

Cooking time: 30 minutes

Servings: 4

Ingredients:

- 2 tablespoons olive oil
- 1 turkey breast, skinless, boneless and cubed
- 1 cup low-sodium beef stock
- 1 cup tomato puree, low sodium
- ¼ teaspoon lime zest, grated
- 1 yellow onion, chopped
- 1 tablespoon sweet paprika
- 1 tablespoon cilantro, chopped
- 2 tablespoons lime juice
- ¼ teaspoon ginger, grated

Directions:

1. Heat up a pot with the oil over medium-high heat, add the onion and the meat and brown for 5 minutes.
2. Add the stock and the other ingredients, bring to a simmer and cook over medium heat for 25 minutes.
3. Divide the mix into bowls and serve for lunch.

Nutrition info per serving: 147 calories, 9.5g protein, 11.1g carbohydrates, 8.1g fat, 2.7g fiber, 18mg cholesterol, 491mg sodium, 488mg potassium

Beef and Beans Salad

Preparation time: 10 minutes

Cooking time: 30 minutes

Servings: 4

Ingredients:

- 1 pound beef stew meat, cut into strips
- 1 tablespoon sage, chopped
- 1 tablespoon olive oil
- A pinch of black pepper
- ½ teaspoon cumin, ground
- 2 cups cherry tomatoes, cubed
- 1 avocado, peeled, pitted and cubed
- 1 cup canned black beans, no-salt-added, drained and rinsed
- ½ cup green onions, chopped
- 2 tablespoons lime juice
- 2 tablespoons balsamic vinegar
- 2 tablespoons cilantro, chopped

Directions:

1. Heat up a pan with the oil over medium-high heat, add the meat and brown for 5 minutes.
2. Add the sage, black pepper and the cumin, toss and cook for 5 minutes more.

3. Add the rest of the ingredients, toss, reduce heat to medium and cook the mix for 20 minutes.
4. Divide the salad into bowls and serve for lunch.

Nutrition info per serving: 533 calories, 47g protein, 39.5g carbohydrates, 21.4g fat, 12.4g fiber, 101mg cholesterol, 88mg sodium, 1686mg potassium

Squash and Peppers Stew

Preparation time: 10 minutes

Cooking time: 20 minutes

Servings: 4

Ingredients:

- 1 pound squash, peeled and roughly cubed
- 1 cup low-sodium chicken stock
- 1 cup canned tomatoes, no-salt-added, crushed
- 1 tablespoon olive oil
- 1 red onion, chopped
- 2 orange sweet peppers, chopped
- ½ cup quinoa
- ½ tablespoon chives, chopped

Directions:

1. Heat up a pot with the oil over medium heat, add the onion, stir and sauté for 2 minutes.
2. Add the squash and the other ingredients, bring to a simmer, and cook for 15 minutes.
3. Stir the stew, divide into bowls and serve for lunch.

Nutrition info per serving: 156 calories, 5.8g protein, 23.7g carbohydrates, 5.2g fat, 4.3g fiber, 0mg cholesterol, 52mg sodium, 601mg potassium

Beef and Cabbage Stew

Preparation time: 10 minutes

Cooking time: 20 minutes

Servings: 4

Ingredients:

- 1 green cabbage head, shredded
- ¼ cup low-sodium beef stock
- 2 tomatoes, cubed
- 2 yellow onions, chopped
- ¾ cup red bell peppers, chopped
- 1 tablespoon olive oil
- 1 pound beef, ground
- ¼ cup cilantro, chopped
- ¼ cup green onions, chopped
- ¼ teaspoon red pepper, crushed

Directions:

1. Heat up a pan with the oil over medium heat, add the meat and the onions, stir and brown for 5 minutes.
2. Add the cabbage and the other ingredients, toss, cook for 15 minutes, divide into bowls and serve for lunch.

Nutrition info per serving: 329 calories, 38.4g protein, 20.1g carbohydrates, 11g fat, 6.9g fiber, 101mg cholesterol, 142mg sodium, 1081mg potassium

Pork Stew

Preparation time: 5 minutes

Cooking time: 8 hours and 10 minutes

Servings: 4

Ingredients:

- 1 pound pork stew meat, cubed
- 1 tablespoon olive oil
- ½ pound green beans, trimmed and halved
- 2 yellow onions, chopped
- 2 garlic cloves, minced
- 2 cups low-sodium beef stock
- 8 ounces tomato sauce, low sodium
- A pinch of black pepper
- A pinch of allspice, ground
- 1 tablespoon rosemary, chopped

Directions:

1. Heat up a pan with the oil over medium-high heat, add the meat, garlic and onion, stir and brown for 10 minutes.
2. Transfer this to a slow cooker, add the other ingredients as well, put the lid on and cook on Low for 8 hours.
3. Divide the stew into bowls and serve.

33

Nutrition info per serving: 357 calories, 38g protein, 16.9g carbohydrates, 14.8g fat, 6.2g fiber, 98mg cholesterol, 587mg sodium, 1139mg potassium

Zucchini Soup

Preparation time: 10 minutes

Cooking time: 20 minutes

Servings: 4

Ingredients:

- 1 tablespoon olive oil
- 1 yellow onion, chopped
- 1 teaspoon ginger, grated
- 1 pound zucchinis, chopped
- 32 ounces low-sodium chicken stock
- 1 cup coconut cream
- 1 tablespoon dill, chopped

Directions:

1. Heat up a pot with the oil over medium heat, add the onion and ginger, stir and cook for 5 minutes.
2. Add the zucchinis and the other ingredients, bring to a simmer and cook over medium heat for 15 minutes.
3. Blend using an immersion blender, divide into bowls and serve.

Nutrition info per serving: 205 calories, 4.2g protein, 10.5g carbohydrates, 18.1g fat, 3.3g fiber, 0mg cholesterol, 151mg sodium, 527mg potassium

Shrimp and Walnuts Salad

Preparation time: 5 minutes

Cooking time: 0 minutes

Servings: 4

Ingredients:

- 2 tablespoons low-fat mayonnaise
- 2 teaspoons chili powder
- A pinch of black pepper
- 1 pound shrimp, cooked, peeled and deveined
- 1 cup red grapes, halved
- ½ cup scallions, chopped
- ¼ cup walnuts, chopped
- 1 tablespoon cilantro, chopped

Directions:

1. In a salad bowl, combine shrimp with the chili powder and the other ingredients, toss and serve for lunch.

Nutrition info per serving: 250 calories, 28.7g protein, 12.9g carbohydrates, 9.2g fat, 1.8g fiber, 241mg cholesterol, 344mg sodium, 369mg potassium

Carrot Soup

Preparation time: 5 minutes

Cooking time: 25 minutes

Servings: 4

Ingredients:

- 2 tablespoons olive oil
- 1 yellow onion, chopped
- 1 pound carrots, peeled and chopped
- 1 teaspoon turmeric powder
- 4 celery stalks, chopped
- 5 cups low-sodium chicken stock
- A pinch of black pepper
- 1 tablespoon cilantro, chopped

Directions:

1. Heat up a pot with the oil over medium heat, add the onion, stir and sauté for 2 minutes.
2. Add the carrots and the other ingredients, bring to a simmer and cook over medium heat for 20 minutes.
3. Blend the soup using an immersion blender, ladle into bowls and serve.

Nutrition info per serving: 128 calories, 2.7g protein, 14.6g carbohydrates, 7.1g fat, 3.8g fiber, 0mg cholesterol, 262mg sodium, 462mg potassium

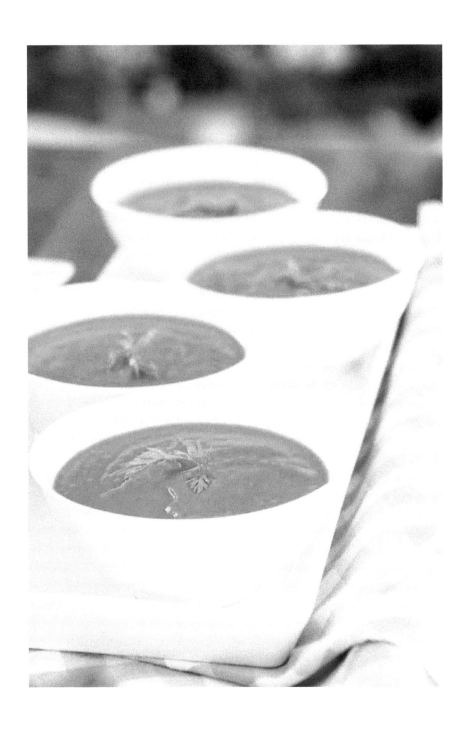

Beef Soup

Preparation time: 10 minutes

Cooking time: 1 hour and 40 minutes

Servings: 4

Ingredients:

- 1 cup canned black beans, no-salt-added and drained
- 7 cups low-sodium beef stock
- 1 green bell pepper, chopped
- 1 tablespoon olive oil
- 1 pound beef stew meat, cubed
- 1 yellow onion, chopped
- 3 garlic cloves, minced
- 1 chili pepper, chopped
- 1 potato, cubed
- A pinch of black pepper
- 1 tablespoon cilantro, chopped

Directions:

1. Heat up a pot with the oil over medium heat, add the onion, garlic and the meat, and brown for 5 minutes.

2. Add the beans and the rest of the ingredients except the cilantro, bring to a simmer and cook over medium heat for 1 hour and 35 minutes.
3. Add the cilantro, ladle the soup into bowls and serve.

Nutrition info per serving: 489 calories, 51.8g protein, 45.1g carbohydrates, 11.4g fat, 9.4g fiber, 101mg cholesterol, 327mg sodium, 1464mg potassium

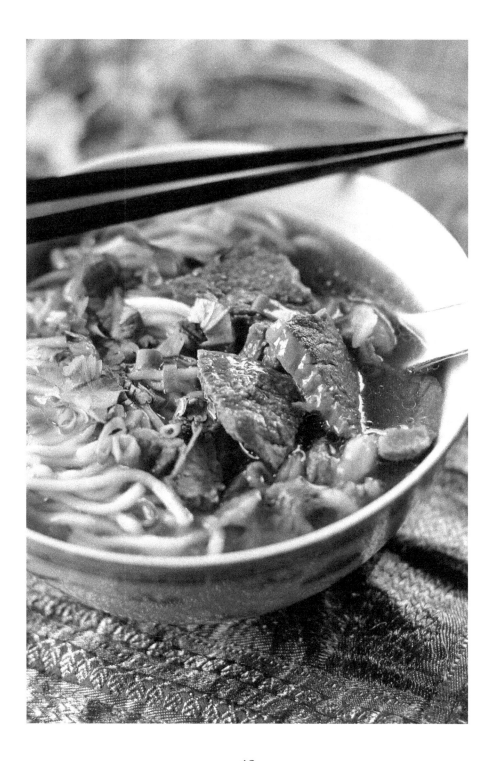

43

43

Salsa Seafood Bowls

Preparation time: 10 minutes

Cooking time: 13 minutes

Servings: 4

Ingredients:

- ½ pound smoked salmon, boneless, skinless and cubed
- ½ pound shrimp, peeled and deveined
- 1 tablespoon olive oil
- 1 red onion, chopped
- ¼ cup tomatoes, cubed
- ½ cup mild salsa
- 2 tablespoons cilantro, chopped

Directions:

1. Heat up a pan with the oil over medium-high heat, add the salmon, toss and cook for 5 minutes.
2. Add the onion, shrimp and the other ingredients, cook for 7 minutes more, divide into bowls and serve.

Nutrition info per serving: 185 calories, 24g protein, 5.3g carbohydrates, 7.1g fat, 0.8g fiber, 132mg cholesterol, 1453mg sodium, 265mg potassium

Chicken and Sauce

Preparation time: 5 minutes

Cooking time: 20 minutes

Servings: 4

Ingredients:

- 1 tablespoon olive oil
- 1 yellow onion, chopped
- A pinch of black pepper
- 1 pound chicken breasts, skinless, boneless and cubed
- 4 garlic cloves, minced
- 1 cup low-sodium chicken stock
- 2 cups coconut cream
- 1 tablespoon basil, chopped
- 1 tablespoon chives, chopped

Directions:

1. Heat up a pan with the oil over medium-high heat, add the garlic, onion and the meat, toss and brown for 5 minutes.
2. Add the stock and the rest of the ingredients, bring to a simmer and cook over medium heat for 15 minutes.
3. Divide the mix between plates and serve.

Nutrition info per serving: 539 calories, 36.3g protein, 10.3g carbohydrates, 40.6g fat, 3.3g fiber, 101mg cholesterol, 151mg sodium, 648mg potassium

Turmeric Chicken Stew

Preparation time: 5 minutes

Cooking time: 20 minutes

Servings: 4

Ingredients:

- 1 pound chicken breasts, skinless, boneless and cubed
- 2 shallots, chopped
- 1 tablespoon olive oil
- 1 eggplant, cubed
- 1 cup canned tomatoes, no-salt-added and crushed
- 1 tablespoon lime juice
- A pinch of black pepper
- ¼ teaspoon ginger, ground
- 1 tablespoon cilantro, chopped

Directions:

1. Heat up a pot with the oil over medium heat, add the shallots and the chicken and brown for 5 minutes.
2. Add the rest of the ingredients, bring to a simmer and cook over medium heat for 15 minutes more.

48

3. Divide into bowls and serve for lunch.

Nutrition info per serving: 286 calories, 34.5g protein, 9.4g carbohydrates, 12.2g fat, 4.6g fiber, 101mg cholesterol, 103mg sodium, 664mg potassium

Chicken Stew

Preparation time: 5 minutes

Cooking time: 20 minutes

Servings: 4

Ingredients:

- 1 pound chicken thighs, boneless, skinless and cubed
- 2 endives, shredded
- 1 cup low-sodium chicken stock
- 1 tablespoon olive oil
- 1 yellow onion, chopped
- 1 carrot, sliced
- 2 garlic cloves, minced
- 8 ounces canned tomatoes, no-salt-added, chopped
- 1 tablespoon chives, chopped

Directions:

1. Heat up a pan with the oil over medium-high heat, add the onion and garlic and sauté for 5 minutes.
2. Add the chicken and brown for 5 minutes more.

3. Add the rest of the ingredients, bring to a simmer, cook for 10 minutes more, divide between plates and serve.

Nutrition info per serving: 279 calories, 34.3g protein, 7.2g carbohydrates, 12.1g fat, 2.1g fiber, 101mg cholesterol, 149mg sodium, 546mg potassium

Turkey and Carrots Soup

Preparation time: 10 minutes

Cooking time: 40 minutes

Servings: 4

Ingredients:

- 1 turkey breast, skinless, boneless, cubed
- 1 tablespoon tomato sauce, no-salt-added
- 1 tablespoon olive oil
- 2 yellow onions, chopped
- 1 quart low-sodium chicken stock
- 1 tablespoon oregano, chopped
- 2 carrots, sliced
- 3 garlic cloves, minced
- A pinch of black pepper

Directions:

1. Heat up a pot with the oil over medium heat, add the onions and the garlic and sauté for 5 minutes.
2. Add the meat and brown it for 5 minutes more.
3. Add the rest of the ingredients, bring to a simmer and cook over medium heat for 30 minutes.
4. Ladle the soup into bowls and serve.

Nutrition info per serving: 79 calories, 2.5g protein, 9.8g carbohydrates, 3.7g fat, 2.5g fiber, 0mg cholesterol, 215mg sodium, 219mg potassium

Cilantro Chicken and Lentils

Preparation time: 10 minutes

Cooking time: 25 minutes

Servings: 4

Ingredients:

- 1 cup canned tomatoes, no-salt-added, chopped
- Black pepper to the taste
- 1 tablespoon chipotle paste
- 1 pound chicken breast, skinless, boneless and cubed
- 2 cups canned lentils, no-salt-added, drained and rinsed
- ½ tablespoon olive oil
- 1 yellow onion, chopped
- 2 tablespoons cilantro, chopped

Directions:

1. Heat up a pan with the oil over medium heat, add the onion and chipotle paste, stir and sauté for 5 minutes.
2. Add the chicken, toss and brown for 5 minutes.

3. Add the rest of the ingredients, toss, cook everything for 15 minutes, divide into bowls and serve.

Nutrition info per serving: 515 calories, 49.8g protein, 63.5g carbohydrates, 6.4g fat, 30.4g fiber, 74mg cholesterol, 112mg sodium, 1486mg potassium

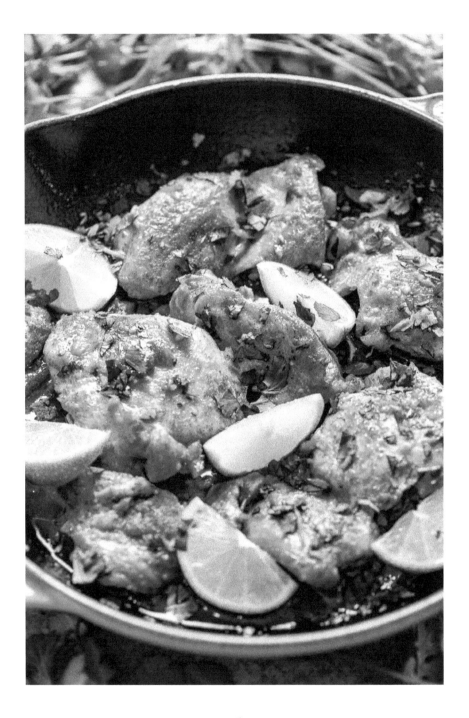

Quinoa Mix

Preparation time: 10 minutes

Cooking time: 20 minutes

Servings: 6

Ingredients:

- 1 red onion, chopped
- 1 tablespoon olive oil
- 15 ounces canned chickpeas, no-salt-added and drained
- 14 ounces coconut milk
- ¼ cup quinoa
- 1 tablespoon ginger, grated
- 2 garlic cloves, minced
- 1 tablespoon turmeric powder
- 1 tablespoon cilantro, chopped

Directions:

1. Heat up a pan with the oil over medium heat, add the onion, stir and sauté for 5 minutes.
2. Add the chickpeas, quinoa and the other ingredients, stir, bring to a simmer and cook for 15 minutes.
3. Divide the mix into bowls and serve for breakfast.

Nutrition info per serving: 472 calories, 16.6g protein, 54.6g carbohydrates, 23g fat, 15.1g fiber, 0mg cholesterol, 29mg sodium, 906mg potassium

.

Peppers Salad

Preparation time: 5 minutes

Cooking time: 15 minutes

Servings: 4

Ingredients:

- 1 cup black olives, pitted and halved
- ½ cup green olives, pitted and halved
- 1 tablespoon olive oil
- 2 scallions, chopped
- 1 red bell pepper, cut into strips
- 1 green bell pepper, cut into strips
- Zest of 1 lime, grated
- Juice of 1 lime
- 1 bunch parsley, chopped
- 1 tomato, chopped

Directions:

1. Heat up a pan with the oil over medium heat, add the scallions, stir and sauté for 2 minutes.
2. Add the olives, peppers and the other ingredients, stir and cook for 13 minutes more.
3. Divide into bowls and serve for breakfast.

Nutrition info per seving: 107 calories, 1.g 7protein, 9.5g carbohydrates, 8g fat, 15.1g fiber, 0mg cholesterol, 376mg sodium, 257mg potassium

Green Beans Hash

Preparation time: 10 minutes

Cooking time: 15 minutes

Servings: 4

Ingredients:

- 1 garlic clove, minced
- 1 red onion, chopped
- 1 tablespoon avocado oil
- 1 pound green beans, trimmed and halved
- 8 eggs, whisked
- 1 tablespoon cilantro, chopped
- A pinch of black pepper

Directions:

1. Heat up a pan with the oil over medium heat, add the onion and the garlic and sauté for 2 minutes.
2. Add the green beans and cook for 2 minutes more.
3. Add the eggs, black pepper and cilantro, toss, spread into the pan and cook for 10 minutes.
4. Divide the mix between plates and serve.

Nutrition info per serving: 178 calories, 13.5g protein, 11.8g carbohydrates, 9.4g fat, 4.6g fiber, 327mg cholesterol, 131mg sodium, 410mg potassium

Eggs Salad

Preparation time: 10 minutes

Cooking time: 0 minutes

Servings: 4

Ingredients:

- 2 carrots, cubed
- 2 green onions, chopped
- 1 bunch of parsley, chopped
- 2 tablespoons olive oil
- 4 eggs, hard boiled, peeled and cubed
- 1 tablespoon balsamic vinegar
- 1 tablespoon chives, chopped
- A pinch of black pepper

Directions:

1. In a bowl, combine the carrots with the eggs and the other ingredients, toss and serve for breakfast.

Nutrition info per serving: 144 calories, 6.4g protein, 4.9g carbohydrates, 11.5g fat, 1.5g fiber, 164mg cholesterol, 92mg sodium, 265mg potassium

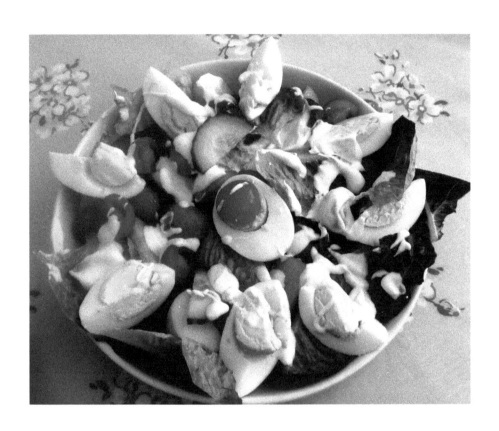

Coconut Berries

Preparation time: 5 minutes

Cooking time: 15 minutes

Servings: 4

Ingredients:

- 3 tablespoons coconut sugar
- 1 cup coconut cream
- 1 cup blueberries
- 1 cup blackberries
- 1 cup strawberries
- 1 teaspoon vanilla extract

Directions:

1. Put the cream in a pot, heat it up over medium heat, add the sugar and the other ingredients, toss, cook for 15 minutes, divide into bowls and serve for breakfast.

Nutrition info per serving: 223 calories, 2.4g protein, 23.9g carbohydrates, 14.7g fat, 4.8g fiber, 0mg cholesterol, 10mg sodium, 301mg potassium

Apples Bowls

Preparation time: 5 minutes

Cooking time: 15 minutes

Servings: 4

Ingredients:

- 1 cup blueberries
- 1 teaspoon cinnamon powder
- 1 and ½ cups almond milk
- ¼ cup raisins
- 2 apples, cored, peeled and cubed
- 1 cup coconut cream

Directions:

1. Put the milk in a pot, bring to a simmer over medium heat, add the berries and the other ingredients, toss, cook for 15 minutes, divide into bowls and serve for breakfast.

Nutrition info per serving: 266 calories, 2.6g protein, 3g14. carbohydrates, 15.6g fat, 5.2g fiber, 0mg cholesterol, 64mg sodium, 373mg potassium

Cinnamon Porridge

Preparation time: 10 minutes

Cooking time: 25 minutes

Servings: 4

Ingredients:

- 1 cup buckwheat
- 3 cups coconut milk
- ½ teaspoon vanilla extract
- 1 tablespoon coconut sugar
- 1 teaspoon ginger powder
- 1 teaspoon cinnamon powder

Directions:

1. Put the milk and the sugar in a pot, bring to a simmer over medium heat, add the buckwheat and the other ingredients, cook for 25 minutes, stirring often, divide into bowls and serve for breakfast.

Nutrition info per serving: 577 calories, 9.8g protein, 44.5g carbohydrates, 44.4g fat, 8.3g fiber, 0mg cholesterol, 36mg sodium, 676mg potassium

Cauliflower Salad

Preparation time: 10 minutes

Cooking time: 20 minutes

Servings: 4

Ingredients:

- 1 pound cauliflower florets
- 1 tablespoon olive oil
- 2 spring onions, chopped
- 1 red bell pepper, sliced
- 1 yellow bell pepper, sliced
- 1 green bell pepper, sliced
- 1 tablespoon cilantro, chopped
- A pinch of black pepper

Directions:

1. Heat up a pan with the oil over medium heat, add the spring onions, stir and sauté for 2 minutes.
2. Add the cauliflower and the other ingredients, toss, cook for 16 minutes, divide into bowls and serve for breakfast.

Nutrition info per serving: 79 calories, 3g protein, 10.8g carbohydrates, 3.7g fat, 4.1g fiber, 0mg cholesterol, 36mg sodium, 430 potassium

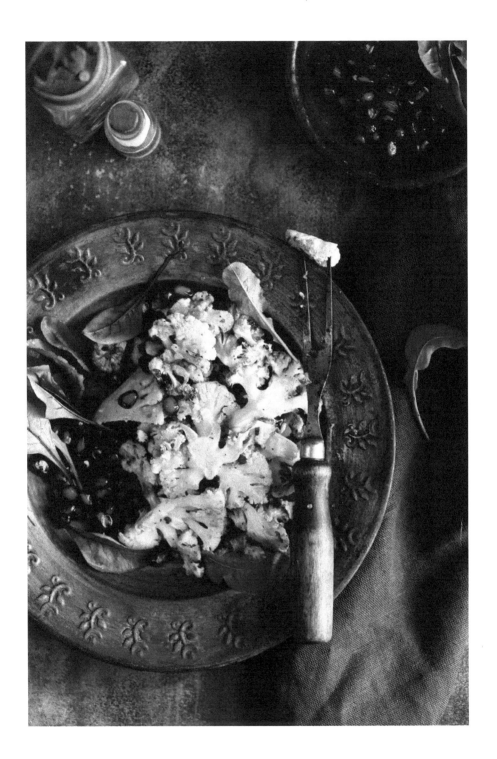

Chicken Hash

Preparation time: 10 minutes

Cooking time: 25 minutes

Servings: 4

Ingredients:

- 2 tablespoons olive oil
- 1 yellow onion, chopped
- 2 garlic cloves, minced
- 1 teaspoon Cajun seasoning
- 8 ounces chicken breast, skinless, boneless and ground
- ½ pound hash browns, low-sodium
- 2 tablespoons veggie stock, no-salt-added
- 1 green bell pepper, chopped

Directions:

1. Heat up a pan with the oil over medium heat, add the onion, garlic and the meat and brown for 5 minutes.
2. Add the hash browns and the other ingredients, stir, and cook over medium heat for 20 minutes stirring often.
3. Divide between plates and serve for breakfast.

Nutrition info per serving: 298 calories, 14.4g protein, 25.2g carbohydrates, 15.6g fat, 2.8g fiber, 36mg cholesterol, 237mg sodium, 639mg potassium

Corn and Beans Tortillas

Preparation time: 5 minutes

Cooking time: 12 minutes

Servings: 4

Ingredients:

- 1 cup canned black beans, no-salt-added, drained and rinsed
- 1 green bell pepper, chopped
- 1 carrots, peeled and grated
- 1 tablespoon olive oil
- 1 red onion, sliced
- ½ cup corn
- 1 cup low-fat cheddar, shredded
- 6 whole wheat tortillas
- 1 cup non-fat yogurt

Directions:

1. Heat up a pan with the oil over medium heat, add the onion and sauté for 2 minutes.
2. Add the beans, carrot, bell pepper and the corn, stir, and cook for 10 minutes more.
3. Arrange the tortillas on a working surface, divide the beans mix on each, also divide the cheese and the yogurt, roll and serve for lunch.

Nutrition info per serving: 478 calories, 24.9g protein, 78.4g carbohydrates, 9.1g fat, 13.8g fiber, 11mg cholesterol, 375mg sodium, 1072mg potassium

Chicken and Spinach Mix

Preparation time: 10 minutes

Cooking time: 20 minutes

Servings: 4

Ingredients:

- 2 chicken breasts, skinless, boneless and cubed
- ¼ cup low-sodium chicken stock
- ½ cup celery, chopped
- 1 cup baby spinach
- 1 mango, peeled, and cubed
- 2 spring onions, chopped
- 1 tablespoon olive oil
- 1 teaspoon thyme, dried
- ¼ teaspoon garlic powder
- A pinch of black pepper

Directions:

1. Heat up a pan with the oil over medium-high heat, add the spring onions and the chicken and brown for 5 minutes.
2. Add the celery and the other ingredients except the spinach, toss and cook for 12 minutes more.

3. Add the spinach, toss, cook for 2-3 minutes, divide everything between plates and serve.

Nutrition info per serving: 227 calories, 22.4g protein, 14.1g carbohydrates, 9.3g fat, 2g fiber, 65mg cholesterol, 89mg sodium, 418mg potassium

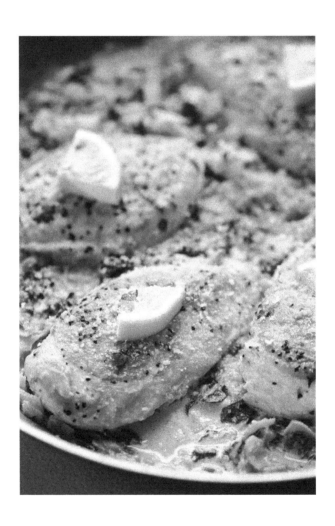

Garlic Chickpeas Fritters

Preparation time: 10 minutes

Cooking time: 10 minutes

Servings: 4

Ingredients:

- 2 garlic cloves, minced
- 15 ounces canned chickpeas, no-salt-added, drained and rinsed
- 1 teaspoon chili powder
- 1 teaspoon cumin, ground
- 1 egg
- 1 tablespoon olive oil
- 1 tablespoon lime juice
- 1 tablespoon lime zest, grated
- 1 tablespoon cilantro, chopped

Directions:

1. In a blender, combine the chickpeas with the garlic and the other ingredients except the egg and pulse well.
2. Shape medium cakes out of this mix.
3. Heat up a pan with the oil over medium-high heat, add the chickpeas cakes, cook for 5

minutes on each side, divide between plates and serve for lunch with a side salad.

Nutrition info per serving: 440 calories, 22.2g protein, 65.9g carbohydrates, 11.3g fat, 19g fiber, 41mg cholesterol, 49mg sodium, 977mg potassium

Cheddar Cauliflower Bowls

Preparation time: 10 minutes

Cooking time: 10 minutes

Servings: 4

Ingredients:

- 1 tablespoon avocado oil
- 1 cup red bell peppers, cubed
- 1 pound cauliflower florets
- 1 red onion, chopped
- 3 tablespoons salsa
- 2 tablespoons low-fat cheddar, shredded
- 2 tablespoons coconut cream

Directions:

1. Heat up a pan with the oil over medium-high heat, add the onion and peppers, and sauté for 2 minutes.
2. Add the cauliflower and the other ingredients, toss, cook for 8 minutes more, divide into bowls and serve.

Nutrition info per serving: 79 calories, 4.4g protein, 12.5g carbohydrates, 2.5g fat, 4.3g fiber, 1mg cholesterol, 134mg sodium, 506mg potassium

Salmon Salad

Preparation time: 5 minutes

Cooking time: 0 minutes

Servings: 4

Ingredients:

- 1 cup canned salmon, drained and flaked, low-sodium
- 1 tablespoon lime zest, grated
- 1 tablespoon lime juice
- 3 tablespoons fat-free yogurt
- 1 cup baby spinach
- 1 teaspoon capers, drained and chopped
- 1 red onion, chopped
- A pinch of black pepper
- 1 tablespoon chives, chopped

Directions:

1. In a bowl, combine the salmon with lime zest, lime juice and the other ingredients, toss and serve cold for lunch.

Nutrition info per serving: 67 calories, 9.2g protein, 4.1g carbohydrates, 1.5g fat, 1g fiber, 21mg cholesterol, 64mg sodium, 245mg potassium

Chicken and Tomato Mix

Preparation time: 10 minutes

Cooking time: 20 minutes

Servings: 4

Ingredients:

- 1 tablespoon olive oil
- 1 pound chicken breast, skinless, boneless and cubed
- ½ pound kale, torn
- 2 cherry tomatoes, halved
- 1 yellow onion, chopped
- ½ cup low-sodium chicken stock
- ¼ cup low-fat mozzarella, shredded

Directions:

1. Heat up a pan with the oil over medium heat, add the chicken and the onion and brown for 5 minutes.
2. Add the kale and the other ingredients except the mozzarella, toss, and cook for 12 minutes more.
3. Sprinkle the cheese on top, cook the mix for 2-3 minutes, divide between plates and serve for lunch.

Nutrition info per serving: 230 calories, 28.2g protein, 11.1g carbohydrates, 7.7g fat, 2.2g fiber, 78mg cholesterol, 158mg sodium, 884mg potassium

Salmon and Olives Salad

Preparation time: 10 minutes

Cooking time: 0 minutes

Servings: 4

Ingredients:

- 6 ounces canned salmon, drained and cubed, low sodium
- 1 tablespoon balsamic vinegar
- 1 tablespoon olive oil
- 2 shallots, chopped
- ½ cup black olives, pitted and halved
- 2 cups baby arugula
- A pinch of black pepper

Directions:

1. In a bowl, combine the salmon with the shallots and the other ingredients, toss and keep in the fridge for 10 minutes before serving for lunch.

Nutrition info per serving: 116 calories, 8.9g protein, 3.1g carbohydrates, 8g fat, 0.7g fiber, 19mg cholesterol, 169mg sodium, 238mg potassium

Shrimp Salad

Preparation time: 5 minutes

Cooking time: 10 minutes

Servings: 4

Ingredients:

- 1 tablespoon olive oil
- 1 pound shrimp, peeled and deveined
- 1 tablespoon basil pesto
- 1 cup baby arugula
- 1 yellow onion, chopped
- 1 cucumber, sliced
- 1 cup carrots, shredded
- 1 tablespoon cilantro, chopped

Directions:

1. Heat up a pan with the oil over medium heat, add the onion and carrots, stir and cook for 3 minutes.
2. Add the shrimp and the other ingredients, toss, cook for 7 minutes more, divide into bowls and serve.

Nutrition info per serving: 200 calories, 27g protein, 9.9g carbohydrates, 5.6g fat, 1.8g fiber, 239mg cholesterol, 300mg sodium, 452mg potassium

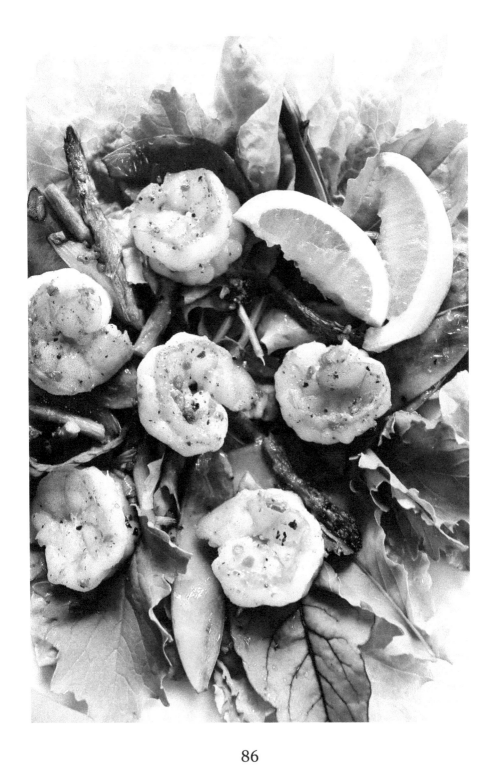

Turkey Tortillas

Preparation time: 10 minutes

Cooking time: 3 minutes

Servings: 2

Ingredients:

- 2 whole wheat tortillas
- 2 teaspoons mustard
- 2 teaspoons mayonnaise, low sodium
- 1 turkey breast, skinless, boneless and cut into strips
- 1 tablespoon olive oil
- 1 red onion, chopped
- 1 red bell peppers, cut into strips
- 1 green bell pepper, cut into strips
- ¼ cup low-fat mozzarella, shredded

Directions:

1. Heat up a pan with the oil over medium heat, add the meat and the onion and brown for 5 minutes
2. Add the peppers, toss and cook for 10 minutes more.
3. Arrange the tortillas on a working surface, divide the turkey mix on each, also divide the

mayo, mustard and the cheese, wrap and serve for lunch.

Nutrition info per serving: 303 calories, 15.9g protein, 37.8g carbohydrates, 11.1g fat, 7g fiber, 15mg cholesterol, 620mg sodium, 394mg potassium

Parsley Green Beans Soup

Preparation time: 5 minutes

Cooking time: 25 minutes

Servings: 4

Ingredients:

- 2 teaspoons olive oil
- 2 garlic cloves, minced
- 1 pound green beans, trimmed and halved
- 1 yellow onion, chopped
- 2 tomatoes, cubed
- 1 teaspoon sweet paprika
- 1 quart low-sodium chicken stock
- 2 tablespoons parsley, chopped

Directions:

1. Heat up a pot with the oil over medium-high heat, add the garlic and the onion, stir and sauté for 5 minutes.
2. Add the green beans and the other ingredients except the parsley, stir, bring to a simmer and cook for 20 minutes.
3. Add the parsley, stir, divide the soup into bowls and serve.

Nutrition info per serving: 87 calories, 4.1g protein, 14g carbohydrates, 2.7g fat, 5.5g fiber, 0mg cholesterol, 147mg sodium, 452mg potassium

Avocado Salad

Preparation time: 5 minutes

Cooking time: 0 minutes

Servings: 4

Ingredients:

- 2 tablespoons balsamic vinegar
- 2 tablespoons mint, chopped
- A pinch of black pepper
- 1 avocado, peeled, pitted and sliced
- 4 cups baby spinach
- 1 cup black olives, pitted and halved
- 1 cucumber, sliced
- 1 tablespoon olive oil

Directions:

1. In a salad bowl, combine the avocado with the spinach and the other ingredients, toss and serve for lunch.

Nutrition info per serving: 192 calories, 2.7g protein, 10.6g carbohydrates, 17.1g fat, 5.7g fiber, 0mg cholesterol, 322mg sodium, 543mg potassium

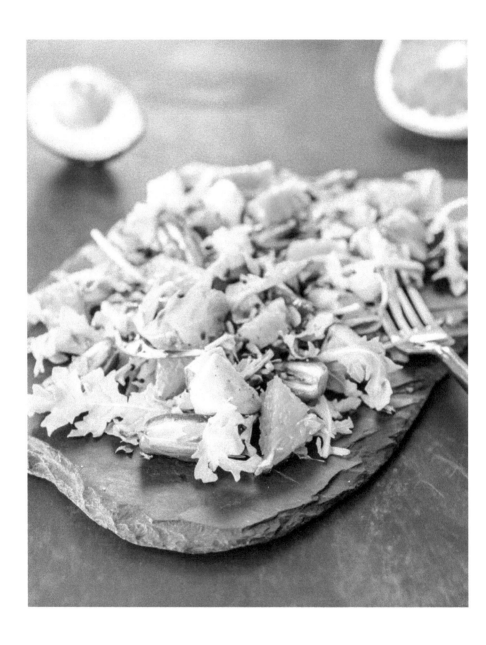

Beef Skillet

Preparation time: 5 minutes

Cooking time: 20 minutes

Servings: 4

Ingredients:

- 1 pound beef, ground
- ½ cup yellow onion, chopped
- 1 tablespoon olive oil
- 1 cup zucchini, cubed
- 2 garlic cloves, minced
- 14 ounces canned tomatoes, no-salt-added, chopped
- 1 teaspoon Italian seasoning
- ¼ cup low-fat parmesan, shredded
- 1 tablespoon chives, chopped
- 1 tablespoon cilantro, chopped

Directions:

1. Heat up a pan with the oil over medium heat, add the garlic, onion and the beef and brown for 5 minutes.
2. Add the rest of the ingredients, toss, cook for 15 minutes more, divide into bowls and serve for lunch.

Nutrition info per serving: 300 calories, 37.2g protein, 9.3g carbohydrates, 12.5g fat, 1.9g fiber, 108mg cholesterol, 184mg sodium, 797mg potassium

Thyme Beef and Tomatoes

Preparation time: 10 minutes

Cooking time: 25 minutes

Servings: 4

Ingredients:

- ½ pound beef, ground
- 3 tablespoons olive oil
- 1 and ¾ pounds red potatoes, peeled and roughly cubed
- 1 yellow onion, chopped
- 2 teaspoons thyme, dried
- 1 cup canned tomatoes, no-salt-added, and chopped
- A pinch of black pepper

Directions:

1. Heat up a pan with the oil over medium-high heat, add the onion and the beef, stir and brown for 5 minutes.
2. Add the potatoes and the rest of the ingredients, toss, bring to a simmer, cook for 20 minutes more, divide into bowls and serve for lunch.

Nutrition info per serving: 355 calories, 21.7g protein, 36.2g carbohydrates, 14.5g fat, 4.7g fiber, 51mg cholesterol, 53mg sodium, 1282mg potassium

Pork Soup

Preparation time: 10 minutes

Cooking time: 25 minutes

Servings: 4

Ingredients:

- 1 tablespoon olive oil
- 1 red onion, chopped
- 1 pound pork stew meat, cubed
- 1 quart low-sodium beef stock
- 1 pound carrots, sliced
- 1 cup tomato puree
- 1 tablespoon cilantro, chopped

Directions:

1. Heat up a pot with the oil over medium-high heat, add the onion and the meat and brown for 5 minutes.
2. Add the rest of the ingredients except the cilantro, bring to a simmer, reduce heat to medium, and boil the soup for 20 minutes.
3. Ladle into bowls and serve for lunch with the cilantro sprinkled on top.

Nutrition info per serving: 354 calories, 36g protein, 19.3g carbohydrates, 14.6g fat, 4.6g fiber, 98mg cholesterol, 199mg sodium, 1104mg potassium

Shrimp and Spinach Salad

Preparation time: 5 minutes

Cooking time: 7 minutes

Servings: 4

Ingredients:

- 1 cup corn
- 1 endive, shredded
- 1 cup baby spinach
- 1 pound shrimp, peeled and deveined
- 2 garlic cloves, minced
- 1 tablespoon lime juice
- 2 cups strawberries, halved
- 2 tablespoons olive oil
- 2 tablespoons balsamic vinegar
- 1 tablespoon cilantro, chopped

Directions:

1. Heat up a pan with the oil over medium-high heat, add the garlic and brown for 1 minute. Add the shrimp and lime juice, toss and cook for 3 minutes on each side.
2. In a salad bowl, combine the shrimp with the corn, endive and the other ingredients, toss and serve for lunch.

Nutrition info per serving: 257 calories, 28g protein, 15.6g carbohydrates, 9.6g fat, 2.9g fiber, 239mg cholesterol, 291mg sodium, 481mg potassium

Raspberry Shrimp and Tomato Salad

Preparation time: 5 minutes

Cooking time: 10 minutes

Servings: 4

Ingredients:

- 1 pound green beans, trimmed and halved
- 2 tablespoons olive oil
- 2 pounds shrimp, peeled and deveined
- 1 tablespoon lemon juice
- 2 cups cherry tomatoes, halved
- ¼ cup raspberry vinegar
- A pinch of black pepper

Directions:

1. Heat up a pan with the oil over medium-high heat, add the shrimp, toss and cook for 2 minutes.
2. Add the green beans and the other ingredients, toss, cook for 8 minutes more, divide into bowls and serve for lunch.

Nutrition info per serving: 379 calories, 53.9g protein, 13g carbohydrates, 11.1g fat, 4g fiber, 478mg cholesterol, 574mg sodium, 613mg potassium

Cod Tacos

Preparation time: 10 minutes

Cooking time: 10 minutes

Servings: 2

Ingredients:

- 4 whole wheat taco shells
- 1 tablespoon light mayonnaise, low sodium
- 1 tablespoon salsa
- 1 tablespoon low-fat mozzarella, shredded
- 1 tablespoon olive oil
- 1 red onion, chopped
- 1 tablespoon cilantro, chopped
- 2 cod fillets, boneless, skinless and cubed
- 1 tablespoon tomato puree

Directions:

1. Heat up a pan with the oil over medium heat, add the onion, stir and cook for 2 minutes.
2. Add the fish and tomato puree, toss gently and cook for 5 minutes more.
3. Spoon this into the taco shells, also divide the mayo, salsa and the cheese and serve for lunch.

Nutrition info per serving: 454 calories, 31.7g protein, 56.1g carbohydrates, 14.5g fat, 7.5g fiber, 38mg cholesterol, 487mg sodium, 142mg potassium

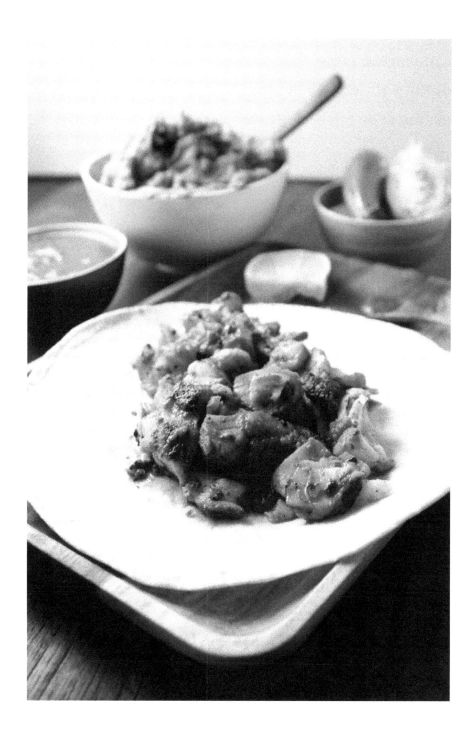

Zucchini Fritters

Preparation time: 10 minutes

Cooking time: 10 minutes

Servings: 4

Ingredients:

- 1 yellow onion, chopped
- 2 zucchinis, grated
- 2 tablespoons almond flour
- 1 egg, whisked
- 1 garlic clove, minced
- A pinch of black pepper
- 1/3 cup carrot, shredded
- 1/3 cup low-fat cheddar, grated
- 1 tablespoon cilantro, chopped
- 1 teaspoon lemon zest, grated
- 2 tablespoons olive oil

Directions:

1. In a bowl, combine the zucchinis with the garlic, onion and the other ingredients except the oil, stir well and shape medium cakes out of this mix.
2. Heat up a pan with the oil over medium-high heat, add the zucchini cakes, cook for 5

minutes on each side, divide between plates and serve with a side salad.

Nutrition info per serving: 204 calories, 8.3g protein, 10.4g carbohydrates, 16g fat, 3.5g fiber, 43mg cholesterol, 96mg sodium, 353mg potassium

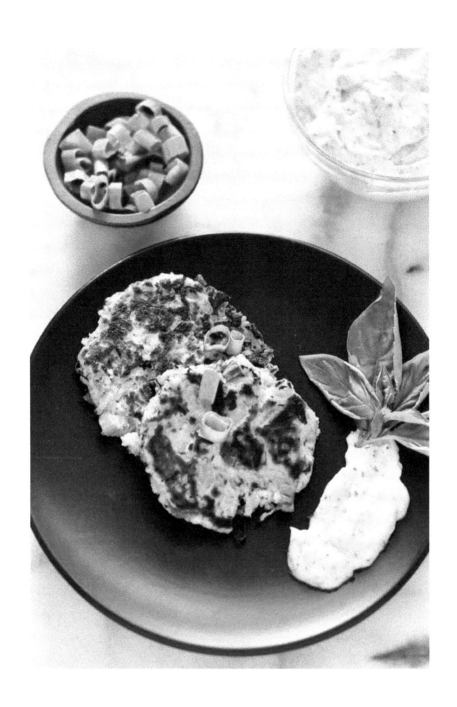